Introduction:

Ketosis is a metabolic condition that changes your body from burning glucose to fat for energy. This change also fuels the brain with energy, owing to the making of ketones in the liver.

Keto diet is a high-fat, low-carb diet, the most strict variation of the LCHF diet (low carb high fat). On a keto diet, the amount of carbohydrates is restricted to 20-28 g per day.
The keto diet is all about decreasing carbohydrate consumption and upping fats. This is to let your body go into the state of ketosis.
A shift your body creates to use fat as a type of energy when it doesn't have sufficient carbs for your cells to use for energy

The Keto Diet is usually a low carb, high fat, modest protein diet. Whenever you eat according to this plan, your metabolism changes to burning stored body fat for energy.
The keto diet has been well known to cut and stabilize blood sugar, advance the overall health and well-being, and cause weight loss.

The keto diet works for several folks who have not had success losing weight in the past.

Though attaining this state of ketosis isn't easy.

To do this, you'll have to follow a very strict diet comprising of fat, protein, and
 almost zero carbs. Moreover, 60 to 80% of your total diet should only consist of fat.

You might consider that adding that much fat to your diet equates to weight gain. As astonishing as it sounds, a Ketogenic diet is ideal for weight loss.

And in addition to weight loss, this fat-based diet also bears lots of other benefits.
Studies show that following a keto diet meal plan could advance
stored fat in demand for fueling.

CHAPTER ONE: Keto Diet FAQ

These are some solutions to some of the most frequent questions about the ketogenic diet.

1. Can I ever eat carbs again?
Yes. Nevertheless, it is essential to eradicate them initially. After the first 2–4 months, you can eat carbs on special occasions — return to the diet instantly after.

2. Will I lose muscle?
There is a bigger risk of losing some muscle on any diet. Moreover, the high protein intake and high ketone levels may help reduce muscle loss, principally if you lift weights.

3. Could you build your muscle on a ketogenic diet?
Yes, moreover, it may not work as well as on a lean-carb diet. More details: Low-Carb/Ketogenic Diets and Exercise routine.

4. Must I have to refeed or carb load?

No. furthermore, a few higher-calorie days, could be beneficial now and then.

5. How much protein must I eat?

Protein should be reasonable, as a very high intake can raise insulin levels and lower ketones. Around 37% of total calorie intake is perhaps the upper limit.

6. What if I am relentlessly tired, weak, or exhausted?

You might not be in total ketosis or be using fats and ketones proficiently. To alter this, reduce your carb intake and re-visit the points above. A supplement similar to MCT oil or ketones may also support it.

7. My urine smells fruity? Why is this?

Don't be worried. This is because of the excretion of byproducts produced during ketosis.

8. My breath smells. What can I do?

This is a common side effect. Try drinking typically flavored water or chewing sugar-free gum.

9. I heard ketosis was extremely dangerous. Is this true?

People regularly mixed ketosis with ketoacidosis. The former is normal, while the latter only happens in unchecked diabetes. Ketoacidosis is dangerous, though the ketosis on a ketogenic diet is entirely normal and healthy.

10. **I have digestion issues and diarrhea. What can I do?**

This common side effect habitually passes after 3–4 weeks. If it lingers, start eating more high-fiber veggies. Magnesium supplements can also assist with constipation.

CHAPTER TWO: A Ketogenic Diet is Splendid, But Not For Everybody

A ketogenic diet can be huge for people who are overweight, diabetic, or looking to improve their metabolic health.

It may be less appropriate for elite athletes or those needing to put together enormous amounts of muscle or weight. However, as with any diet, it will only work if you are unfailing and stay with it in the long-term.

That being said, somethings are as well established in nutrition as the potent health and weight loss benefits of a ketogenic diet.

Switching to butter and bacon to lose weight and further health might not scream "winning plan" to everyone. However, it makes good sense to those on the ketogenic diet (or "keto diet"), the newest "it" routine that backs high-fat, moderate-protein, and low-carbohydrate eating.

Of course, behind every healthy diet, there's controversy. Amid the criticisms of
 the keto diet, cynics say the plan is too limiting, lacks nutritional balance, and hasn't been considered for long-term effects (the keto diet ranked 39th out of 40 for Best Diets Overall 2018 by a U.S. News report).

On a joking side, others—involving some medical experts—plan a well-formulated keto diet is sustainable and meets necessary nutrient needs; they also point to
 increasing research linking the diet to potential health benefits.

Though it may be new to you, the keto diet has been around since the 1920s, when
the Mayo Clinic revealed its effectiveness for assisting epilepsy (that is still the case).

 Since then, there's definite proof that the keto diet assists with weight loss including type 2 diabetes, prediabetes, and metabolic syndrome, states Jeff Volek, Ph.D., RD, a professor in the Department of Human Sciences at The Florida State University

What Is a Genuine Ketogenic Diet?

On a ketogenic diet, you're usually eating a diet that's high in fat (roughly 71 percent of your total calories is from fat), moderate in protein (about 19percent of your calories), and low in carbohydrate (about 4 percent of calories).

By limiting carbohydrates (to habitually less than 46 grams for the average person), your body lacks the glucose (from carbs)

that is, in general, uses for energy, so it ultimately switches over to burning fat as its primary fuel source instead; throughout a metabolic process termed ketosis,
the liver converts the fat into fragments of fatty acids termed ketones, which control the brain and other organs and tissues.

Everyone has to get their nutritional sweetened spot for making abundant ketones and staying in ketosis, however "the core

system of the diet is to sustain carbohydrate intake low enough, so your body continues producing ketones at high levels," states Volek.
"Your body gets this alternative fuel and becomes very capable at breaking down and burning fat.".

Who Ought Not To Be on the Keto Diet?

Blanket statement: It's often the best to check with your physician before starting

on this regimen. With that understanding, "the keto diet isn't good for persons with liver or kidney disease, or somebody with a medical condition,

similar to a gastrointestinal issue, who can't make use of high quantities of dietary fat," states Sarah Jadin, a Los-Angeles licensed dietitian and originator of Keto Consulting,
If you've had your gallbladder eliminated, the keto diet might be a no-go. '

Women who are pregnant or breastfeeding and folks with some rare genetic problems shouldn't try this diet.
"When you're using the keto diet for medical nutrition therapy, you require

medical oversight to be successful," implies Jadin. "Moreover, anyone thinking the keto diet would benefit from consulting with a medical expert, similar to a dietitian, who is well-versed in this diet."

CHAPTER THREE:

Ketogenic Diet Other Advantages

Positive science on ketosis, along with personal successes conveyed by word-of-mouth, has driven more people to discover the ketogenic diet, states Volek. At present, the keto diet tries to have an assuring therapeutic role in cancer, Alzheimer's, Parkinson's, and polycystic ovary syndrome (PCOS).

The study is still premature in several areas, but Volek suspects there will more definitive answers in the broader scope of the diet's benefits within the next decade.

Benefit #1: Weight Loss

You may experience quick weight loss in the first week due to fluid loss, but then after a few weeks, you'll probably notice more pounds peeling away.

Many causes for this weight loss are being looked at; however, the journal Obesity Reviews, shows that ketosis subdues your appetite, which squashes the desire to eat.

Benefit #2: Control Blood Sugar
Most carbs you eat are broken down into sugar that gets the bloodstream. When you take in carbohydrates on the keto diet, you have lower levels of blood glucose (high blood glucose can lead to diabetes).

A study in the journal Nutrition shows that a ketogenic diet improves blood glucose levels in people with type 2 diabetes more considerably than a low-calorie diet and can also decrease the dosage of your diabetes meds.

Benefit #3: Enhance Cholesterol and Blood Pressure
A consideration of various studies in the journal Nutrients found that ketogenic diets are associated with major reductions in overall cholesterol, rises in "good"
HDL cholesterol levels, dips in triglycerides levels and decreases in "bad" LDL cholesterol;
There are some salient questions as to whether diets high in saturated fat go against these benefits.
The same paper states that a ketogenic may somewhat reduce blood pressure, but science is still minimal on this point.

Benefit #4: Lower Inflammation
With inflammation contributing to most chronic diseases, the keto diet is anti-inflammatory and may assist relieve some inflammation-connected pain
 conditions, according to researchers at Trinity College. One mechanism at play:
The keto diet reduces sugar and processed foods that can lead to oxidative trauma in the body, a reason for chronic inflammation.
Benefit #5: Longer Life
This might be more of a maybe, but new studies on mice fed a ketogenic diet lived

much longer, coming from Cell Metabolism. "Not only did these mice live much longer, but they also had extended health in terms of physical and cognitive functioning," says Volek. "Meaning, they lived happy, healthy lives." clearly, human studies need to be performed.

Other Side Effects of Keto Diet

You can have an entirely smooth transition into ketosis, or…not. As your body is adjusting to using ketones as your new fuel source, you might experience a variety of uncomfortable short-term symptoms.

These signs are known as "the keto flu." Low-sodium levels are always to blame for symptoms keto flu since the kidneys secrete more sodium when you're in ketosis, says Volek. A few side effects:

Headache and Dizziness
Most folks on the keto diet have to bump up their daily salt intake by an extra gram or two to prevent side effects like headaches, dizziness, and even fainting, says Volek. To get rid of the symptoms caused by salt depletion,
Volek proposes drinking broth made with a bouillon cube (which has somewhat less than 1 gram of sodium), once or twice a day.
Constipation
When you consume a high-fat diet, you slow down your gastric emptying, and your motility, which could lead you to constipation, states Jadin.

Making sure you're having that extra bit of sodium, consuming enough fiber-filled non-starchy vegetables, and drinking ample fluids (as you urinate more on the keto diet) can move things along.

Heart Palpitations

When you're deficient sodium, your kidney may wind up releasing potassium, and you could as well end up with a mineral instability that leads to problems with your heartbeat, explains Volek.

Optimal Ketosis and Macros

Achieving optimal ketosis depend on getting the proper balance of macronutrients (or "macros" in keto-speak); these are the constituent in your diet that account for the more significant part of your calories, a.k.a. Energy—precisely, fat, protein, and carbohydrates.

By the way, it's always "net grams" of carbohydrates that are counted toward your daily intake; "net" reduces the amount of fiber in a food from its carbohydrate total.

To know you're spot-on diet-wise (given that the macros mix that launch you into ketosis varies between persons),
you can gauge ketones in your blood (with a finger prick kit) or more generally, through your urine (cheaper, but not as accurate).

Instinctively, the way you think can also serve as a guide to whether you're in ketosis. Most people on ketosis are more emotionally sharp and energized, and feel less hungry.

The amount you should eat is dependent on several factors, similar to your weight, gender, and activity levels. Online keto calculators can do the mathematics for you.

Supplements You Can Take:
Take a multivitamin. "Because you are eliminating grains, the bulk of fruits, some vegetables, and a major amount of dairy from your menu, a multivitamin is good insurance against any micronutrient deficiencies," says Jadin.

Depending on what your individual in general diet looks like, expert means you might also require to add extra calcium, vitamin D, and potassium supplement.

Many supplement their keto diets with quality MCT oil (MCT goes for medium-chain triglycerides). Jadin's opinion:

It may assist boost ketosis, but it's not essential, and some people can't stand the supplement.

CHAPTER FOUR: Sample Ketogenic Menu Plan:

Regulate these meal ideas to meet your individual needs on the keto diet.

Monday

1. Breakfast: spinach omelet with bacon
2. Lunch: leafy green salad put together with salmon and oil-based dressing
3. Dinner: a lettuce-wrapped burger with spicy mayo

Tuesday

1. Breakfast: flaxseed porridge with blueberries and cinnamon
2. Lunch: egg salad poached with avocado
3. Dinner: baked turkey meatballs parmesan topped with zucchini noodles

Wednesday

1. Breakfast: egg, cheddar, pepper "breakfast mini-muffins."

2. Lunch: Sautéed cheese on keto bread (home-grown or keto-friendly store-bought bread) with enough salad

3. Dinner: Tofu roasted in sesame oil with vegetables

Thursday

1. Breakfast: keto smoothie (with an EXCELLENT avocado base, and later a combo of greens, nuts, berries, and a little heavy cream)

2. Lunch: tuna salad mixed celery stalks

3. Dinner: sausage- and veggie-poached pizza on cauliflower pizza crust

Friday

1. Breakfast: eggs wrapped with cheddar and tomatoes

2. Lunch: chicken salad lettuce wrap

3. Dinner: steak cooked in butter with asparagus

Saturday

1. Breakfast: vanilla chia pudding

2. Lunch: crust-less bacon, mushroom, swiss quiche

3. Dinner: lamb chops with Brussels sprouts

Sunday

1. Breakfast: fried eggs chopped bacon and avocado chopped

2. Lunch: Fried chicken with stir -fry broccoli and cauliflower

3. Dinner: Taco salad with good ground beef, guac, and sour cream (with no shell)
What Is The Keto Diet?

The keto diet (also recognized as a ketogenic diet, low carb diet, and LCHF diet) is a low carbohydrate, high-fat diet. Sustaining this diet is an immense tool for weight loss.
 More significantly, though, from an increasing number of studies, it helps reduce risk factors for diabetes, heart diseases, stroke, Alzheimer's, epilepsy, and more.

On the keto diet, your body gets into a metabolic state termed ketosis. When in ketosis, your body is making use of ketone bodies for energy in place of glucose.
Ketone bodies are gotten from fat and are a much more stable, steady source of energy than glucose, which is derived from carbohydrates.

Getting into ketosis generally takes anywhere from 4 days to a week. As soon as you're in ketosis, you'll be using fat for energy in place of carbs. This shows the fat you eat and stored body fat.

Testing For Ketosis:

You can conduct the test yourself to see whether you've gone into ketosis just a few days after you've started the keto diet! Make use of a ketone test strip, and it will give you the level of ketone bodies in your urine.

If the concentration is high enough, you've effectively entered ketosis! *Note: Any change to the strip color shows that you are in ketosis.*

There are other ways of knowing you're in ketosis, though – look for changes in your mood and attentiveness, as well as a stronger smell in your breath and urine.
Many persons also report better sleep and reduced enthusiasm when they're in ketosis.

The Truth About Fat

You could be thinking, "that eating a lot of fat is horrendous!" The truth is, many studies and meta-studies with over 920,000 subjects

have arrived at comparable conclusions: Consuming saturated and monounsaturated fats have no effects on heart disease risks.
Most fats are good and are necessary for our health. Lipids (fatty acids) and protein (amino acids) are vital for survival.

Fats are the most effective form of energy, and each gram has about 10calories, as compared to 5calories per gram of protein and carbohydrates.
There is no such thing as a necessary carbohydrate.

The keto diet encourages eating fresh, whole foods similar to meat, fish, veggies, and healthy fats and oils as well as significantly reducing processed and chemically treated foods the Standard American Diet (SAD) has so long encouraged.

It's a diet that you can maintain long-term and adore. What's not to relish about bacon and eggs in the morning?

Calories & Macronutrients

How Calories Work:

A calorie is a unit of energy. When something contains 200 calories, it shows how much energy your body could get from ingesting it. Calorie consumption dictates weight gain/loss.

If you burn an average of 1,900 calories and eat 2,020 calories per day, you will gain weight.

If you do some exercise that uses an extra 355 calories per day, you'll use 2,120 calories per day, putting you at a disadvantage of 100 calories.

Only by eating at a deficit, you will lose weight because your body will tap into stored resources for the outstanding energy it needs.

That being said, it's vital to get the right balance of macronutrients every day so your body has the energy it requires.

What Are Good Macronutrients?

Macronutrients (macros) are elements that our bodies use to produce energy for themselves – majorly fat, protein, and carbs. They are positioned in all food and are measured in grams (g) on nutrition labels.

- **Fat** gives 9 calories per gram
- **Protein** offers 4 calories per gram
- **Carbs** give 4 calories per gram

Net Carbs

Several low carb recipes will write "net carbs" when showing their macros. Net carbs are total carbs subtracted from dietary fiber and sugar alcohols.

Our bodies couldn't break down fiber and sugar alcohol into glucose, so they usually don't raise blood sugar. For this reason, many persons on a low carb diet don't count them toward their total carb count.

How Much Should You Eat?

On a keto diet, about 67 to 77 percent of the calories you consume daily should come from fat. About 22 to 32 percent ought to come from protein. The remaining 6 percent or so should come from carbohydrates.

You could use our Keto Diet Calculator to figure out precisely how many calories and which macros you ought to be eating daily!

It questions you for basic info like your weight, activity levels, and goals and immediately gives you the quantities of fat, protein, and carbs you might be eating each day.

Carbs: What precisely Are They?

Carbohydrates (carbs) are a macronutrient gotten in things like starches, grains, and foods high in sugar. This comprises, however, isn't restricted to, bread, flour, rice, pasta, beans, potatoes, sugar, syrup, cereals, fruits, bagels, and soda.

Carbs are broken down into glucose (a kind of sugar) in our bodies for energy. Eating any kind of carbs spikes blood sugar levels. The spike may occur faster or slower depending on the type of carb (simple or complex), but the peak will still happen.

Blood sugar spikes cause stable insulin releases to battle the spikes. Constant insulin gives results in fat storage and insulin resistance.
 After many years, this cycle often leads to prediabetes, metabolic syndrome, and also type 2 diabetes.
In a full of sugar, cereal, pasta, burgers, and large sodas, you could see how carbs can be overconsumed.

Where We Are Today?

According to the 2016 report by the Centers for Diseases Control and Prevention (CDC), more than 1 in 7 grown up in the U.S. (88 million people) have prediabetes, a state in which blood glucose is habitually high and frequently leads to type 2 diabetes and many other medical problems.

Today, almost 1 in 15 persons in the U.S. have type 2 diabetes compared to nearly 1 in 40 in 1982. Fat has been liable as the bad guy and companies have been producing low-fat

and fat-free, chemically-laden alternatives of almost every type of food in existence.
Nevertheless, obesity, diabetes, and heart disease rates are also increasing.
Almost 1 in 15 adults in the U.S. has type 2 diabetes, nearly 4 times more than 32 years ago.

Fat is Making a Comeback

We're starting to comprehend that carbs in large quantities are much more harmful than previously thought, while most fats are healthy and essential.

The nutritional landscape is altering.
Ketogenic diet and low carb diet collections, as well as similar dietary clusters like paleo, are growing, and a nutritional revolution is beginning. We are starting to value the detrimental effects of our relationship with excess sugar and carbs.

CHAPTER FIVE: Long-Term Benefits

Studies continuously show that those who eat a low carb, high fat diet rather than a high carb, low-fat diet:
- Eliminate more weight and body fat
- Have good levels of good cholesterol (HDL and large LDL)
- Have lessened blood sugar and insulin resistance (majorly reversing prediabetes and type 2 diabetes)20,21
- Experience a reduction in craving
- Have lessened triglyceride levels (fat molecules in the blood that lead to heart disease)
- Have considerable reductions in blood pressure, leading to a reduction in heart disease and stroke24

Eating a keto/low carb diet makes you lose more weight than eating low fat.

Day-to-Day Benefits

The keto diet doesn't only offer long-term advantages! Whenever you're on keto, you could expect to:
- Lose body fat

- Have steady energy levels in the course of the day
- Stay very satisfied after meals longer, with reduce snacking and overeating

Longer satiation and consistent energy levels are as a result of the majority of calories coming from fat, which is slower to assimilate and calorically denser.

Being on a low carb diet also reduces blood glucose spikes and crashes. You won't have swift blood sugar drops leaving you feeling weak and bewildered.

Entering Ketosis:

The keto diet's main aim is to put you in nutritional ketosis all of the time. If you're about getting started with your keto diet, you should eat up to 27 grams of carbs per day.

When you're in ketosis for long enough (about 4 to 9 weeks), you grow into keto-improve or fat-adapted. This is when your glycogen lessens (the glucose stored in muscles and liver), you convey less water weight, muscle endurance increases, and your general energy levels are higher.

Another advantage of being keto-modified is that you can eat ~50 grams of net carbs a day to maintain ketosis.

Type 1 Diabetes & Ketoacidosis

If you have type 1 diabetes, check with your doctor before starting a keto diet. Diabetic ketoacidosis (DKA) is a risky condition that can occur if you have type 1 diabetes due to a shortage of insulin.

Avoiding The Keto Flu

What is Keto Flu?
The keto flu usually happens to keto dieters due to low levels of sodium and electrolytes and has flu-like symptoms, including:
- Fatigue
- Headaches
- Cough
- Sniffles
- Irritability

- Nausea

It's significant to note that this isn't the real flu! It's termed keto flu due to similar symptoms, but it is not at all contagious and doesn't involve a virus.

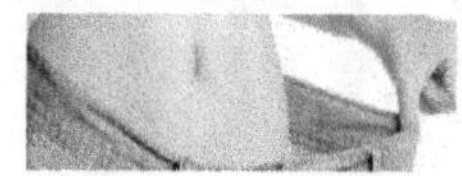

Why Does It Happen?

The primary source of keto flu is your deficient body electrolytes, specifically sodium. When beginning keto, you cut out lots of treated foods and eat more whole, natural foods. Though this is great, it causes an unexpected drop in sodium intake.

Besides, dipping carbs reduces insulin levels, which reduces sodium stored by kidneys.

Between your reduced sodium consumption and stored sodium flushed by your kidneys, you end up being low on sodium and other electrolytes.
The keto flu can be eliminated by consuming enough electrolytes, mainly sodium.

Ending the Keto Flu:

The best way to shun (or end) the keto flu is to add more sodium and electrolytes to your diet. These are the most effective (and tasty) ways to get more sodium:
- Adding more salt to your food
- Drinking soup broth
- Eating ample of salty foods similar to bacon and marinated vegetables

Attempt to eat more sodium as you start the keto diet to thwart the keto flu completely. If you do catch it, remember that it'll go away quickly and you'll emerge a fat-burning machine.

Is the keto diet safe?

Specialists are divided on whether the keto diet is a good idea.
Furthermore, Lori Chang,
a registered dietitian and a counselor at the Center for Healthy Living at Kaiser Permanente West Los Angeles starts using a "cleaner" source of energy—ketones rather

than quick-burning carbohydrates—can enhance mood and energy levels.

When you ingest refined carbohydrates or just too many carbs in general, the blood is flooded with excess insulin, Chang says.

"This could lead to a blood sugar rollercoaster that stresses the body and negatively impacts energy levels and mood.

When you're in a state of ketosis, moreover, ketone bodies don't need insulin to cross the blood-brain barrier, which wards off unsustainable blood sugar levels."

Other professionals say the long-term accumulation of ketones could be damaging. "Those ketones are back up fuel bases, and we're not used to running on them long-term," says Kristen Kizer, a qualified dietitian at Houston Anglican Hospital.

"Ketones are negatively-charged molecules, which are known to be acidic.

Whenever you build up ketone bodies in your system, you're building up acid. One of the techniques your body safeguards acid is by drawing calcium from your bones.

" Kizer also states that the diet isn't very balanced and has a very high intake of animal products, which usually do not guard against cancer, diabetes, or other diseases.

When you do try the diet outside of medical supervision, the expert says it's essential to examine your urine with urinalysis ketone test strips to guarantee your ketone levels don't become seriously high.

Ketone urine test strips also make use of by individuals with diabetes to know if they're at risk for ketoacidosis (DKA), a life-threatening problem that occurs when an individual doesn't have enough insulin in their body.

(Healthy ketosis is well-thought-out to be 0.5 to 3.0 mM blood ketones.)

:

CHAPTER Six: 5 -ingredients ketogenic recipes that anyone can cook

1 BLT Chicken Stuffed Avocados [The Garlic Diaries]

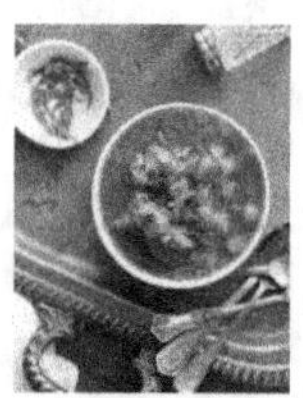

It is crammed with a flavor combining ingredients such as turkey bacon, rotisserie chicken, Roma tomatoes, cottage cheese, green lettuce, and, clearly, avocados! If you haven't tried this sautéed avocado recipe, let me tell you are missing a lot!

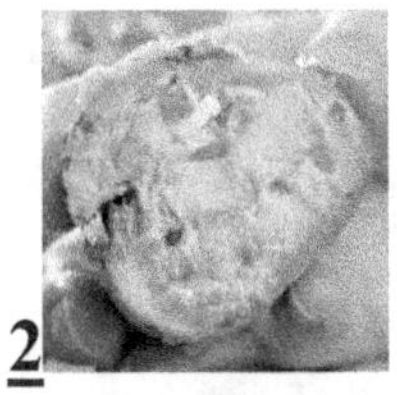

`Chipotle Added with Pork Lettuce Wraps With Avocado Aioli [Fashionable Foods] Making use of remaining delicious slow cooker chipotle pulled pork; all these keto recipe needs is topping lettuce wraps and topping with avocado! The Aioli is super easy too!

3 Cheddar-Topped Taco Rolls [Wicked sautéed] Keto, grain-free taco rolls are just like burritos, short of the carbs! The "crust" is based on the cheddar cheese, and the rest is the perfect mixture of spicy taco meat, tomatoes, and avocado.

4 Vegetarian Keto Club Salad [Ruled. Me] **Are you** looking for vegan keto diet recipes for lunch? Give this one a try! Though

cheddar cheese, romaine lettuce, cherry tomatoes, diced cucumbers, hard-boiled eggs, and savory spicing dressing, this vegetarian salad will keep you nourished and filled all through the day.

5 Avocado Egg Salad, Avocado egg salad, is mayo-free made from crunchy bacon, dill, green onions, lime juice, cheese, and some yogurts!

6 Vegan Crack Slaw For a worthy vegetarian keto lunch, Go for this vegan mode of the known crack slaw recipe created with green cabbage and macadamia nuts. Spicy with chili paste, sesame oil, garlic oil, and green onions, this recipe is just too special!

7 **<u>Fresh Tuna Salad Recipe</u> [Nancy Ferrer]** Packed with healthy fats, this fresh tuna salad would not sadden you! Created from tuna, Roma tomatoes, cucumbers, purple onions, a fraction mayo, and a fraction of sea salt, this tuna salad is one of my greatest clean ingestion keto diet recipes!

8 Spicy Thai Chicken Zoodle Soup [Fantastic Foods] Tasty and healthy routine to get your vegetables! Besides, it only takes 32 minutes total to prepare!

9 Fresh Sriracha Broccoli Salad [Wicked Stuffed] fantastic way to stay full for lunch! This broccoli salad is as spicy as it looks with fresh broccoli, red peppers, cheddar cheese, sunflower seeds, and bacon.

10 Caprese Hasselback Chicken with [Low Carb Maven] Makes this tremendous Hasselback chicken with mozzarella, Roma tomatoes, fresh basil, sesame oil, and balsamic vinegar in less than 32 minutes! One of our major keto diet recipes by all standards!

11 Slow Cooker Chipotle Pulled Pork [Fashionable Foods] packed with flavor and super easy! Use the snippets for a range of keto diet recipes similar to Chipotle sautéed Pork Lettuce topped!

12 Sheet Pan Roasted Asparagus & Chicken With Chorizo [Eat Drink &Paleo] This sheet pan meal comes handy in over 32 minutes, making use of chicken, asparagus, and pleasant herbs and spices.

13 Easy Cashew Chicken If you don't have a lot of time, but you are hungry for a home-cooked meal, try this Easy Cashew Chicken that comes together in 17 minutes!
The exceptional Keto Bacon and Egg Cups Recipe
14 Bacon, Bacon and More Bacon
This is devoted to the outstanding "Keto Bacon and Egg Cups" recipe on the web. Though, before we give you the delightful secrets about this recipe, let's step back for a minute.
You might not believe me, but there is an enormous amount of yummy advantages to being on a ketogenic diet.

And one of those advantages is eating lots of sweet, sweet bacon. We've known about bacon "dangers," as it can cause high cholesterol, but no one ever seems to mention the benefits.

For instance, did you know that bacon indeed contains omega-3 fatty acids, which are the same nutrients found in fish? And it's these particular fatty acids that *help* guard the heart and keep it functioning correctly. Bacon also has a lot of a nutrient named choline.

This nutrient is mostly vital for memory, and native intelligence and scientists have even found it could assist fight off mental impairments such as Alzheimer's disease. Amazing, right?
Thus, at the moment, we've revealed the benefits of bacon; let's go on to the recipe.

Recipe Advantages:
What you should know about this exceptional recipe, is that it's full of the all-essential protein keto dieters require.

This is not only because of the lack of sugary carbohydrates but because it's main ingredients are bacon (you guessed it!), eggs, and cheese.

And merely to let you know, it's very much impossible to discover three parts that contain as much protein as these.
Hence, for anyone trying to get their fat intake up, while protecting their other macros down, these little cups are perfect.

We propose eating these for breakfast, as they're straightforward to make. For illustration, there are only four steps to the whole recipe,
while our last step is just a top tip to review how to cook the eggs precisely as you like them.

They're also perfect as a protein-filled snack if you're having an above all ravenous morning or evening.

Even though they take 27 minutes to prepare, twenty minutes of that is cooking time! Result! When you're often in a bit of a rush, though, feel free to cook these in multiples and freeze them.

It would save you so much time that you can then spend on more vital activities, similar to caring for your kids or having extra leisure time! Be cautious if you like to recook these, moreover.
Make sure they have completely defrosted and are piping hot when taking them out of the oven.

You could check the temperature with a kitchen utensil and don't burn yourself by eating them instantly.

Nutritional Information:

Now for the stats. This keto bacon and egg cups have 212 calories per cup, and you're getting 16 grams of protein and 16 grams of fat. Even better, it only has zero carbs, which is just unbelievable for keto!
It also makes them ideal for anyone who has dietary intolerances and is, for example, gluten-free.
So, what are you waiting for! All you need is seven minutes of your time to cook this dish,

And then you could have a tasty, ketogenic snack, breakfast, or brunch any time you wish. Wonderful? We think so too.
<<Nutritional Info is 'Per Cup'>>

Steps
 1

This recipe could not be more natural, and would have you in bacon and egg heaven before you know it! First up, get a suitable tray and grease with a little oil to thwart the bacon and eggs from sticking.

2

Optional If, love us, you adore your bacon on the crispy side; you can fry up your bacon in a pan for some minutes before you put it in the tray.

3

Place one slice of bacon into each muffin slot; confirm that the bacon is topped about the sides and not at the bottom of the tin.

4

Break an egg into each hole of the bacon. Spray a little salt and pepper on top and top it off with a sprinkling of your chosen grated cheese (we could use sharp cheddar).

5

Put these bad boys in the cooker for 24 minutes at 352 degrees F (180 C). When they surface, they will be bubbling with keto goodness. I relish to eat these hot or cold, and always take cold ones to work for a snack in my lunchbox. A great little meal for boosting your fat intake!

6

TOP TIP If you desire your eggs a bit more runny, cook the bacon inside the muffin tin for 12 minutes first, and then crack in the eggs before cooking for another 10.

15 Breakfast Porridge
– Paleo Flourish

Ingredients: Almonds, coconut cream, sweetener of your choice, cinnamon powder, nutmeg, cloves, cardamom.
Perfect for the colder mornings, this porridge is ideal for the whole family. If you favor your oatmeal sweeter, then we propose you add in a dash of stevia. The cinnamon and cloves provide a warm aroma to this breakfast dish.
16 Natural Nut and Seed Keto Granola
– Paleo thrive

Ingredients: almonds, cashews, pumpkin seeds, chia seeds, cacao nibs, coconut flakes. Avocado

This granola is so simple to make as all you do is mix the constituents! It could be stored like other granolas, but because it does not contain oats,

it is possible to cause fewer inflammatory problems, and it cuts out more carbs.

17 Creamy Shrimp and Bacon skillet

– The Nourished Caveman

Ingredients: uncured organic bacon, mushrooms, Roasted salmon, shrimp, coconut cream, sea salt, ground black pepper.

This is a beautiful combination of flavor and texture.

The cream can be swapped with coconut cream if you are dairy-intolerant. This meal can be indeed frozen, so it is best for cooking in batches, so you habitually have something spicy in the freezer.

This could be served over zucchini noodles but tastes great on its own.

18 Dijon Pork Breakfast Skillet

– Holistically Engineered

Ingredients: ground pork, mushrooms, zucchini, green pepper, garlic powder, sea salt, basil, broccoli,Dijon mustard.

This is quite a filling breakfast, nevertheless full of flavor! It has heat from the mustard and added meatiness from the mushrooms.

This is a one-pot recipe, so it doesn't necessitate much washing-up. If you ingest eggs, then this dish would taste good with an egg on top, though it is tasty just on its own.

19 Breakfast Sausage
– Cook Eat Paleo

Ingredients: pork, sage, burned sweet paprika, smoked hot paprika, sea salt, ground pepper.

These sausage patties take only some minutes to plan and can be frozen, so why not get ready a bigger batch and use them up later?

This is a very flexible recipe since you can use spices of your own choice. Even though pork and sage are great partners, you could also add some chili to spice things up. Or try putting some rosemary in place.

20 Almond Cereal

– Pencils and Pancakes

Ingredients: almonds, fry pumpkin seeds, chia seeds, coconut milk, water, blueberries.

Keto breakfast cereal recipes, just like this one, are best in the morning as they give you an excellent base to carry you throughout a busy morning.

Cook them in advance for a super swift breakfast.

21 Corned Beef Hash

– Wholly cooked

Ingredients: corned beef, red onion, radishes, garlic, beef broth, salt, pepper.

This is a breakfast dish that is packed with flavor. When you are not sure about getting radishes, let us support you that cooking them makes a much mellower flavor.

You could also add in some remaining cabbage if you have it. Garlic and onion are such an ideal blend, and they go so well with corned beef. This is a brilliant way to get your protein and veggies in.

22 Ketogenic Breakfast Smoothie

– Paleo Flourish

Constituents: spinach, almonds, brazil nuts, coconut milk, greens powder.

If you have never made use of green smoothies, then this is a grand opening. So swift and easy to make, this is a perfect standby for a busy morning as it takes only five minutes to organize.

The use of the nuts gives great extra flavor to the smoothie. It can be hard to get enough vegetables and fiber into your keto diet, so keep some greens powder handy in your kitchen.

23 Low Carb Strawberry Crunch Smoothie

—

Ingredients: unsweetened vanilla almond milk, cheese strawberries, cinnamon, almonds, chia seeds (not compulsory).

This smoothie is so yummy that even children will relish it! There can't be many persons who don't like strawberries, and with the putting of the almonds and chia seeds, this is a revealing way to start the day.

Fruits are sweet, so you won't need to add any other sweetener, and the cinnamon, which studies show is useful for controlling blood sugars, makes this smoothie extra tasty.

CHAPTER SEVEN: Best Keto Diet Recipes – Appetizers

24 Buffalo Chicken Wings Recipe
– Paleo Flourish

Constituents: chicken wings, coconut flour, cayenne pepper, black pepper, red pepper flakes, paprika, garlic powder, salt, ghee, and hot sauce

These are distinct for festivals, dinner parties, or for an easy adult lunch.

With the heat applied to this pepper, these wings are spicy! After putting them together, put them back in the refrigerator for 33 minutes, and that should help the coating to stick better.

25Chicken & Bacon Nibbles with Green Onion & Sage
– Meatified

Ingredients: includes bacon, ground chicken, green onion, ground sage, garlic powder
Putting bacon to these little bites will guarantee they are never dried out as some burgers can be.
Attempt to use the best bacon you can get as it adds to the flavor and by making use of green onions offers this dish a herbal hint.

26Tuna Poke Avocado Boats
– Anya's Eats

Ingredients: tuna, coconut amino, grilled sesame oil, cucumber, macadamia nuts, black sesame seeds (non-compulsory), avocados.
This recipe makes use of raw tuna, so make sure to purchase sushi-grade tuna.
These boats look special. So create them for dinner parties or special events.

27 Cream of Celery Soup
– Forest and Fauna
Ingredients: contains celery, yellow onion, coconut milk, water, dill, sea salt.

A delicious and nutritious soup, this handy recipe could be cooked on a stove or in a soup maker. In place of adding water to thin the soup,

You ought to add vegetable broth to make the recipe appropriate for vegans. Or make use of chicken broth, which goes undoubtedly well with the celery.

28 Kale Guacamole
– Savory Lotus

Ingredients: composed of kale, white onion, red avocados, cilantro, garlic, sea salt, lime juice, cumin.

The kale and avocados in this favorite dish are filled full of nutrients, antioxidants, and vitamins.

This dish makes an excellent dip for veggies or a topping for burgers. The cilantro and lime offer such freshness to the bowl and help to cut through the creamy texture of the avocado.

29 Sardine Pate
–

Ingredients: Compose of butter, sardines, shallot, green onion, parsley, lemon juice, Dijon-style mustard, salt, pepper, parsley.

A swift and easy recipe to prepare, yet it makes a beautiful beginner to a dinner party! Sardines have such a strong flavor on their own; however,
this is settled by serving them with cucumber slices or celery sticks to increase freshness.

Ahi Tuna Ceviche with Sesame and Mint 30 Crispy Garlic Curry Chicken Drumsticks Recipe
– Paleo Flourish

 Ingredients: It contains chicken drumsticks, salt, curry powder, garlic powder, coconut oil
These astonishing drumsticks take only six minutes to prepare.
The curry flavor has been `a tasty for many some years and is even alluring to the kids. If you wish to guarantee that the coating on these drumsticks is crunchy, then make sure the meat is dry by tapping it with a kitchen cloth.

31 Grilled Chicken Drumsticks with Garlic Marinade
– Paleo Flourish

 Ingredients: it contains chicken drumsticks, olive oil, garlic, lemon, sea salt, pepper

If you could, marinade the chicken in this recipe for at least two hours before putting them on the grill.

These juicy and tender drumsticks are often a favorite, particularly with the kids who find it thrilling to be able to put food in their hands!

32 Easy Mediterranean Chicken
– The Healthy Foodie

Ingredients: it contains chicken breasts, dried oregano, smoked paprika, salt, pepper, bell peppers, tomatoes, jalapeño peppers, green onions, lime.

The blend of flavors and colors from the peppers and tomatoes in this dish makes it look so attractive!

The spices bring a genuine Mediterranean taste to this recipe. Moreover, you could push out the jalapenos if you are not too ready for the heat.

33 Oven-Fried Chicken
-Everyday Maven

Ingredients: composed of chicken, almond meal, blanched almond flour, salt, black pepper, cayenne pepper, paprika, dried oregano, garlic powder, eggs, almond milk, sesame oil.

Lemon juice has long been spicy to serve with chicken, hence try this recipe for your next dinner party!

The dish has a pretty smokey hint from the paprika, and you can save the juices to make as a sauce over the chicken instantly it is cooked. One excellent option is to serve up this with a green salad of your choice.

34 Chicken Shawarma

– Paleo Cupboard

Ingredients: chicken thighs (or its breasts), extra virgin olive oil, lemon juice, sea salt, ground black pepper, dried thyme, paprika, turmeric, allspice, garlic powder, onion powder, cinnamon, and cayenne pepper.

Shawarma is known to cooking on an open spit and shaving off the meat when it is cooked; however, this tastes just as good cooked in a grill.

The whole family will relish these, whether for a primary meal or if you are grilling outside for family and friends.

The blend of spice gives this dish a stunning result – memorize to soak the skewers in water first when you are using wooden ones to avoid them burning.

35 Easy Pan-Fried Lemon Chicken

– Stupid Easy Paleo

Ingredients: chicken breast, lemon, olive oil or heated coconut oil, sea salt, and black pepper.

To make sure that the flavors all join with the chicken, try to marinate the meat for at least 30 minutes. The marinade causes the beef to uphold its tenderness and keeps the chicken juicy. If you are taking the dish with lemon zest, try to use the most exceptional grater setting you can.

36 Easy 5-Ingredient Baked Mustard Chicken

– Kokopaleo

Ingredients: coconut oil, chicken breasts, peppery brown mustard, and almond meal/flour

This dish is excellent for someone with a busy schedule because it's so easy to make.

There is a latent heat in this tasty dish that comes from using the mustard to coat the chicken, though milder mustard could be used if this is being served to children. Serve with your good choice of salad leaves to guarantee you get ample of veggies into your ketogenic diet.

37 Chicken Puttanesca
– DJ Foodie

Ingredients: extra virgin olive oil, chicken breasts, garlic, red onion, Italian olives, capers, anchovy filets, red chili flakes, tomatoes, salt, and pepper

This recipe is a delight on a traditional Italian dish and makes excellent use of olives and garlic, two of Italy's most natural ingredients.

Although this is an astonishing meal, you might be a little put off by the use of anchovies. Don't panic! It is relatively easy to use sliced bacon in its place to add a bit of smokiness.

You could also leave the chili flakes if you don't like the heat.

Best Keto Recipes – Beef Entrees

38 Easy Zucchini Beef Sautee with Garlic and Cilantro
– Paleo Flourish

Ingredient: Beef, zucchini, cilantro, garlic, gluten-free tamari sauce, avocado, or coconut oil or garlic oil

This recipe is very stress- free and swift to make. Because you include zucchini into this dish, it does not need any accompaniment, but if you love, it could be served with cauliflower rice.
It's ideal for a quick ketogenic dinner at the end of your day.
39 Quick Ground Beef Stir-Fry
– Paleo Flourish

 Ingredients: ground beef, green bell peppers, tomatoes, white onion, garlic, cilantro, hot sauce, salt, pepper, coconut oil.
This is a swift and stress-free ketogenic recipe which is so resourceful. It offers you with a warming and tasty meal in a short time.

 If you would instead not use the vegetables itemized in this recipe, then miss them out and use your favorites or leftovers. If you are not sure of using hot sauce, then you can ignore it or use a dash.

40 Bacon Cabbage Chuck Beef Stew
– The Nourished Caveman

Ingredients: compose of Bacon, roast, red onions, garlic, cabbage, sea salt, black pepper, thyme, beef bone consommé.

Everyone has a passion for a dish like this on a cold day. This beef stew is marvelous and full of taste. As this is a steady cooker recipe, the making of it is straightforward.
It's a perfect meal to come home to after a hard day's work. If you are not too joyful about using thyme, then you could try using another herb of your choice.

41 Spicy Beef Curry
– That Paleo Couple
Ingredients: comprises of Beef, white onion, curry powder, garlic, ginger, full-fat coconut milk, salt, chili sauce.
This is a tasty beef curry recipe using onion, garlic, and ginger as its base.

If you are using chuck steak, which could be a little tight, permit the curry to rest some minutes immediately, serving to re-marinate the meat. Appreciate this curry by itself for a keto dinner or over cauliflower rice.

42 Meaty Chili
– Swiss Paleo
Ingredients: Ground beef, chicken sausages, chili powder, cumin, dried oregano,

cinnamon, tomatoes, tomato paste, onions, Anaheim peppers, poblano pepper, green olives, garlic, sea salt, red pepper.

Chili is a special dish that is very common with the whole family. This dish typically has beans in it, but you can also benefit from bean-less chili on the ketogenic diet (seeds are high in carbs).
If you do not love the chili to be too spicy, then you could serve it with avocado, which would take down the heat.

43 Spicy Jalapeno Burgers
– Paleo in Practice

Ingredients: ground beef, jalapeño pepper, ground cumin, ground garlic, red pepper flakes, onion, salt, pepper.
These highly spiced burgers make an excellent addition if you are grilling outside, or merely for a family meal.
The cumin and garlic give the beef an extensive boost in flavor and make them a trendy choice.

If you are eager to cook in batches, these burgers can be frozen uncooked and kept for another day. If you are refrigerating these, it is a nice idea to separate them with sheets of greaseproof paper first so that you could divide them more effortlessly.

Best Keto Recipes – Pork Entrees

44 Pork Spare Ribs Recipe
– Paleo Flourish

Ingredients: pork spare ribs (or back ribs), ginger, scallions, star anise, Szechuan peppercorns, garlic, gluten-free tamari sauce, extra virgin coconut oil, salt (optional).

This is founded on a traditional Chinese recipe, but without using any of the usual sugary ingredients associated with Chinese take-out. Once the ribs are boiled, you could sieve the broth and re-use it as a base for soups.
Ginger comes into many of Chinese recipes and adds a subtle kick; however, fresh ginger is so much better than powdered! It can be frozen too, so grate off what you require, then put it back in the freezer.

45 Easy Collard Greens With Bacon
– Meatified

Ingredients: Bacon, onion, bacon fat or walnuts oil with sesame oil, white onion, garlic, collard greens, chicken stock, apple cider vinegar.

This is a stress -free way of using up collard greens that you might have in your freezer.

Combine them with the bacon, and you got a beautiful dish that can be used as a side for other good dishes or as the main one.

The apple cider vinegar put a little zest that helps take away any resentment from the greens.

46 New Mexico Carne Avocado

– She Cooks He Cleans

Ingredients: it contains Pork, New Mexican chilies, chicken or beef stock, onion, garlic, Mexican oregano, ground cumin, ground coriander, kosher salt, pepper apple cider vinegar.

This dish meets the bit of extra time it takes to prepare, as the finished result is astonishing! You can change the strength of chills you use to make this recipe a bit more palatable for the whole family.

For instance, use ancho chills if you want a milder flavor. The pork ends up so soft and full of flavor! Attempt serving it with a salad or with topped tomatoes, or use avocado to cool it down even more.

47 Chili Verde
– Fit and Fresh
Ingredients: coconut oil, pork shoulder, garlic, onion, chicken stock, tomatillos, jalapeños, cumin, red pepper flakes, salt, pepper, cilantro, limes.

Using a slow cooker for this sort of recipe can be a perfect solution for someone who has a hectic life. It cooks long and slow whenever you are at work.
Through the addition of the salsa, the pork is tender and delicious. If you do not adore cilantro, make sure you used flat-leaf parsley instead.

48 Ginger Pork with Broccoli
– Fed and Fit
Ingredients: butter, pork chops, Celtic sea salt, ground black pepper, garlic powder, ginger powder, coconut aminos, lime juice, fish pasty, broccoli, cilantro leaves, red pepper flakes, lime slices.

This is another recipe with its roots in Chinese cooking. Pork and ginger is a usual combination which goes well with the broccoli to produce a lovely dish. To give the chops a crispy look and since they are not coated, cook them in batches slowly – patience is needed to attain the best results!

49 Stir-Fried Pork with Cabbage Noodles sautéed Chicken Skewers Recipe with Garlic Sauce [Paleo, Keto, AIP]

As the summer approaches, firing up the top is a brilliant option for creating fast and delicious meals.
These meshed chicken skewers are easy to make, and the garlic sauce is just delicious with it.

STEP 1: Heat the grill to high. Thus, using wooden skewers, soak them in water first. For the Garlic Sauce, put the garlic cover and salt inside the blender. Then add in around 1/6 cup of the lemon juice and 1/2 cup of olive oil.

STEP 2: Blend well for 5-11 seconds, then slow your blender down and sprinkle in more lemon juice and olive oil on the other hand until you hear the blender sound shift a bit (it's subtle!).

The paste will then change into mayo-like consistency. If it doesn't work, don't bother – the sauce won't look astonishing, though it'll still taste good!

STEP 3: Retain half the garlic sauce to serve with. Take the other half of the garlic spits and add in the extra 1/2 cup of olive oil and teaspoon of salt. Mix well – this produces the marinade.

STEP 4: cut the chicken, onion, bell peppers, and zucchini into roughly 1-inch cubes or squares. Mix them in a container with the marinade.

STEP 5: Place the cubes on spits and chop on high till the chicken is cooked (typically, we grate on the bottom for a few minutes to get the charred look and then move the spits to a top rack with the lid down to cook the chicken well).

STEP 6: Serve it with the garlic paste you reserved.

Ingredients
For the Skewers
- 1 lb chicken breast, chopped into large cubes (roughly. 1-inch)
- 1 onion, sliced
- 2 bell peppers, chopped (omit for AIP)
- 1 zucchini

For the Garlic Sauce
- 1 head garlic, skinned
- 1 teaspoon salt
- Approx. ¼ cup lemon juice
- Approx. 1 cup olive oil

Additional requirements for the marinade
- ½ cup olive oil
- 1 teaspoon salt

Instructions

1. Heat the grill to high. If using wooden skewers, immerse them in water first. For the Garlic Sauce, put the garlic cloves and salt into the blender. Then put in around 1/6 cup of the lemon juice and 1/2 cup of olive oil.

2. Mix well for 5-10 seconds, then slow your blender down and drizzle in more lemon juice and olive oil otherwise until you hear the blender sound shift a bit (it's subtle!).
The consistency will then change into a mayo-like texture. If it doesn't work, don't bother – the sauce won't look astonishing, though it'll still taste good!

3. Preserve half the garlic sauce to serve with. Take the other half of the garlic paste and add in the extra 1/2 cup of olive oil and teaspoon of salt. Mix well – this makes the marinade.

4. Slice the chicken, onion, bell peppers, and zucchini into roughly 1-inch cubes or squares. Mix them in a vessel with the cooked one.
5. Place the cubes on spits and chopped on high up until the chicken is cooked (typically, we sliced on the bottom for a few minutes to get the charred appear and then transfer the skewers to an upper rack with the lid down to boil the chicken well).
6. Serve with the garlic sauce you set aside.

Notes

TIP: Making an emulsion (that mayo -like a paste) can be tough if you're new to it, so don't be concerned too much if it looks a bit ugly. It still tastes good.

All nutritional data are projected and based on per serving amounts.
Nutrition
- **Serving Size:** 1 large plate
- **Calories:** 580
- **Sugar:** 1 g
- **Fat:** 33 g
- **Carbohydrates:** 11 g
- **Fiber:** 2 g
- **Protein:** 55 g

50 Get the Recipe: Creamy Tuscan Garlic Chicken

Dish this hospitable-quality chicken dish over rice or pasta to round out your meal.
Prep Time
11 minutes
Cook Time
16 minutes
Difficulty
easy
Servings
5
Ingredients
- 1 1/3 lbs boneless skinless chicken parts, chopped into cutlets

- 2 tablespoons olive oil
- Salt and pepper, to taste
- 1 cup heavy cream
- 1/2 cup chicken broth
- 1 teaspoon garlic powder
- 1 teaspoon Italian seasoning
- 1/2 cup parmesan cheese
- 1 cup spinach, chopped
- 1/2 cup sun-dried tomatoes

Instructions

1) Season chicken with salt and heated pepper, then heat in a large skillet on medium-high heat for 4-6minutes on each side, until browned and comprehensively cooked. Set chicken aside on a plate.

2) Bring the heat down to medium. In the same skillet, put in the heavy cream, chicken broth, garlic powder, Italian seasoning, and parmesan cheese for some minutes until the mixture thickens to some extent.

3) Add spinach and sundried tomatoes. Boil for a minute or two, until spinach wilts. Return chicken to the pan and flip a few times, so that it is carefully coated in sauce.

51 Loaded Cauliflower (low carb, keto)

This healthy, packed cauliflower tastes just like full potato skins short of all the carbs. Made with butter, sour cream, chives, cheddar cheese, and bacon, it's the definitive side for keto diets.

Some weeks ago, I brought you lovely folks one of my favorite recipes for pounded cauliflower with celery root and spoke about how cauliflower is the superman of the low carb world.
We use it for nearly everything, don't we?

I know that I've individually roasted cauliflower with bacon and green onions as a side and have pureed it to add more body to the cream of celery soup. I've also flavored it with exotic Indian spices in a superb vegetable masala, and I've added it to the hearty beef curry.

One of my favorite ways to relish cauliflower is as cauliflower fritters that *sub for hash browns*. Yum!

Even conventional bloggers have known cauliflower and are making great cauliflower pizzas like this one from Kevin at Closet Cooking. And Lisa from Low Carb Yum makes use of cauliflower in some of her desserts – chocolate pudding anyone?
Loaded Cauliflower Recipe
You could see that cauliflower can be utilized for nearly any dish. Though you, my low carb faithful's, already know this. You've been cauliflower devotees for years!

For me, it's the more easy recipes that hit home – such as this **loaded cauliflower mash**. It's the *ultimate in comfort food.*

If you were one who liked ordering loaded potato skins at Friday's after work or favored a completely baked potato with your steak, this recipe would remind you of the days. At least, it happened to me!

And those who relished twice-baked potatoes need not give an old favorite since this healthy low carb cauliflower feels so good, I could have termed it twice baked cauliflower casserole!
The tip to getting a fluffy cauliflower mash:

1. Steam instead of boil.
2. let it sit exposed to discharge some moisture
3. Dry it well just before putting it in the food processor
4. Put the ingredients that make it taste great – like *sour cream, cheddar cheese, chives, and bacon.*

That's it. Comfortable, cheesy, and lovely!
My kids couldn't get enough.
These are die-hard crushed potato haters!
This healthy complete cauliflower was a hit in every recipe book and a win for me!

 Loaded Cauliflower (low carb, keto)
This full cauliflower, made with butter, sour cream, chives, cheddar cheese, and bacon, is the ultimate in little carb comfort food!
Course Side Dish
Cuisine American
Keyword bacon, cauliflower, cheese
Prep Time 11 minutes
Cook Time 11 minutes
Total Time 22 minutes
Servings 4 people
Calories 300kcal

Ingredients

- 2-pound cauliflower
- 4 ounces sour cream
- 1 cup peeved cheddar cheese
- Two slices bacon boiled and crumbled
- 2 tablespoons chives sliced
- 3 tablespoons butter
- 1/4 teaspoon garlic powder
- salt and pepper to taste

Instructions

1. Sliced the cauliflower into florets and put them to a microwave-safe bowl. Put 2 tablespoons of water and cover with cling film. Microwave for 5-9 minutes, reliant on your microwave, until wholly cooked and tender.

Drain the excess water and let sit exposed for a minute or two.

(Alternately, steam your cauliflower the orthodox way. You might require squeezing a little water out of the cauliflower after cooking.)

1. Put the cauliflower to a food processor and process until fluffy. Place the butter, garlic powder, and sour cream and process until it resembles the consistency of mashed potatoes. Eliminate the mashed cauliflower to a bowl and add most of the chives, saving

some to add to the top later. Place half of the cheddar cheese and blend by hand. Spice it with salt and pepper.

2. Topped the loaded cauliflower with the remaining cheese, outstanding chives, and bacon. Put back into the microwave to dissolve the cheese or put the cauliflower under the broiler for a few minutes.
3.   **Serves 5 people at 4.7g Net Carbs.**
NOTE: When making ahead and refrigerating, I find it best to microwave at 52% power for some minutes to take the chill off before placing it in the microwave oven to finish warming up and then placing under the broiler.

This will freeze, however, replace the sour cream with cream cheese instead.

Nutrition
Calories: 300kcal | Carbohydrates: 7.5g | Protein: 11.7g | Fat: 24.7g | Saturated Fat: 15.6g | Polyunsaturated Fat: 0.8g | Monounsaturated Fat: 5g | Cholesterol: 76mg | Sodium: 286mg | Potassium: 379mg | Fiber: 4g | Sugar: 4.85g

52 Creamy Cauliflower Mac and Cheese Casserole with Hamburger

Roasted Cauliflower With Bacon and Caramelized Green Onion

The impeccable Low Carb Mashed Potatoes

Keto Cheese Shell Taco Cups

The Keto Cheese Shell Taco Cups is the stress-free way to get your taco on…low carb style!
Raise your hand if you adore tacos.
I can tell how many hands are raised right at the moment and how many of you are so thrilled about this recipe.

Well, in between the craziness of moving and being 39 weeks pregnant, my innovative plan didn't quite work out
But I'm still really enthusiastic about showing you the latest innovation in low carb taco-eating.
53 Keto Cheese Shell Taco Cups

Keto Cheese Shell Taco Cups

Ingredients
cheese cups
- 7–9 slices of Colby jack cheese, or preferred cheese

salsa
- 2 Roma tomatoes, diced
- 3 tbsp diced the red onion
- 1/2 fresh jalapeno, diced superbly
- Juice from a lime
- 3 tbsp cilantro

other, optional
- Tart cream, taco meat of high-quality, avocado, etc

Instructions
1. Preheat oven to 376
2. Put wedges of cheese on the parchment-lined baking sheet with some inches in between slices
3. Bake for about 6 minutes or until bubbly and just beginning to brown at edges
4. Eradicate baking sheet and let cool a couple of minutes
5. Carefully pick up slices and place in the muffin tin to form a cup shape, let cool extra 10 minutes

Salsa

1. Put Roma tomatoes, onions, jalapeno, lime juice, and cilantro in a medium enclosed vessel in the fridge for at least 33 minutes, or serve instantly -it gets more flavorful the longer it is in the refrigerator

Assemble cups by filling with favored fillings and enjoy

Salmon seasoned with a tasty Cajun spice mix and pan-fried until crispy served capped with refreshing and creamy avocado salsa!

54 Blackened Salmon with Avocado Salsa Preparation Time: 7 minutes **Cook Time**: 15 minutes Complete **Time**:18 minutes **Servings**: 5

Salmon seasoned with a delicious cajun spice blend and pan-fried until crispy served topped with refreshing and creamy avocado salsa!

Ingredients

For the blackened salmon:
- 1 tablespoon oil
- 4 (6 ounces) pieces salmon
- 4 teaspoons Cajun seasoning

For the avocado salsa:

- 2 avocado, diced
- 1/4 cup red onion, diced
- 1 jalapeno, superbly diced
- 1 tablespoon cilantro, chopped
- 1 tablespoon lime juice
- salt to taste

For the avocado and cucumber salsa:
- 2 avocado, diced
- 1 cup cucumber, diced
- 1/4 cup green onion, diced
- 1 tablespoon parsley, sliced
- 1 tablespoon lemon juice
- salt to taste

Directions

For the blackened salmon:

1. Heat the oil in a huge bottom skillet over medium-high heat, add the salmon, seasoned with the Cajun seasoning, and cook until extremely golden brown to somewhat blackened before flipping and repeating for the other side.

For the avocado salsa:

1. Mix everything and enjoy the salmon!

For the avocado and cucumber salsa:

1. Mix everything and revel in the salmon!

Option: Use trout, tilapia, or other fish in place of salmon.

Note: Offer the salmon with one of the avocado salsa or the avocado and cucumber salsa.

Nutrition Facts: Calories 446, Fat 31.3g (Saturated 5.8g, Trans 0), Cholesterol 76mg, Sodium 72mg, Carbs 9.9g (Fiber 7.2g, Sugars 2.0g), Protein 36.1g
Nutrition by:

55 Roasted Lemon Butter Garlic Shrimp and Asparagus

ONE PAN Roasted Lemon Garlic Butter Shrimp and Asparagus blended with chili flakes, and fresh parsley is not only packed with flavor
but on your table in 16MINUTES! No joke! This recipe is the most refreshing, most satisfying meal that tastes downright gourmet.

Stock enough frozen shrimp, and you could make this lavish tasting meal at a moment's notice. Place the (customizable heat) curried lemon garlic butter shrimp plain or make it into lemon garlic butter shrimp pasta!

Prep Time
11 minutes

Cook Time
12 minutes

Servings
-6 servings

Ingredients
Asparagus
- 1 pound thin/medium asparagus ends trimmed
- 1 tablespoon olive oil
- 1 garlic clove, minced
- 1/4 teaspoon salt
- 1/8 teaspoon pepper

Shrimp
- 2 1/2 pounds medium unprepared skinned shrimp deveined*
- 1 tablespoon olive oil
- 2-3 garlic cloves, minced
- 1/3 teaspoon salt
- 1/4 teaspoon paprika
- 1/8 teaspoon pepper
- 1/8-1/4 teaspoon red pepper flakes

- 3 tablespoons topped fresh parsley
- 2 1/2 tablespoons lemon juice or more to taste
- 3 tablespoons butter, cubed

Serve with

- Pasta
- Rice

Instructions

1. Preheat oven to almost 400 degrees F.
2. Stroke a Jelly Roll Pan (10x16) with foil and lightly spray with cooking spray.
Put asparagus and sprinkle with 2 tablespoons olive oil. Put 2 sliced garlic clove, 1/4 teaspoon salt, and 1/8 teaspoon pepper. Toss until habitually coated then line asparagus in a single layer — roast for 4-7 minutes dependent on thickness.

3. In the meantime, remove tails from shrimp.

4. Remove pan from the cooker and push asparagus to one side of the pan (keep in a single layer). Put shrimp and sprinkle it with 2 tablespoons olive oil. Put 2-4 crushed garlic cloves (or more to taste), 1/2 teaspoon salt, 1/6 teaspoon paprika, 1/8 teaspoon pepper,

1/8-1/4 teaspoon red chili flakes and new parsley. Toss till evenly coated then line shrimp in a single layer.

5. Top asparagus with 2tablespoon cubed butter, evenly spaced. Top shrimp with 2 tablespoons cubed butter, well-spaced. Roast for 7 minutes or just until shrimp is opaque.

6. Eliminate pan from oven and drizzle with lemon juice. Season with extra salt and pepper to taste serve with pasta, rice, etc.

56 Keto Chicken Enchilada Bowl
I created this Keto Chicken Enchilada Bowl on the stovetop, but it could be made in a cooker or an Instant Pot by adding the chicken, enchilada sauce, chilies, and onions together and allowing them to cook on low heat all day.

The chicken and sauce blend could ALSO be planned ahead of time and frozen, so when it's time to reheat
(I would possibly let it thaw and then heat in a pot on the stovetop), you can add a steamer bag of cauliflower rice and your fresh toppings. Pretty simple!

Another alternative would be to make the cauliflower yourself. If you're not used to the dish, it's pretty simple, just grated cauliflower that you can prepare yourself with a new head and a food processor. My new favorite way to make it is found in my Keto Mexican Cauliflower Rice recipe. Delicious!

57 Easy Keto Chocolate Fudge

Nutrition Info

Nutrition
- **Serving Size:** 1/4 recipe yield
- **Calories:** 568 Calories
- **Fat:** 40.22g
- **Carbohydrates:** 6.13g NET Carbs
- **Protein:** 38.39g

Hands-on 11 minutes Overall 22 minutes
Nutritional values (per serving)
Net carbs3.3 grams
Protein38.8 grams
Fat43.9 grams
Calories 582 kcal
Calories from carbs **3%**, protein **29%**, fat **71%**
Total carbs**10.6**grams**Fiber7.5** grams

Total carbs**10.6** gramsFiber**7.5** gramsSugars**1.3** grams   Saturated fat**10.2** gramsSodium**533** mg(23% RDA)Magnesium**80** mg(20% RDA)Potassium**1,032** mg(52% EMR)

Here's a breakdown of the nutrition. The recipe has been improved to make the complete recipe more flawless.

For 1/5 of this recipe we're going for :

Calories: 569Calories
Total Carbs: 10.42g
Fiber: 4.28g
Net Carbs: 6.16g
Protein: 38.39g
Fat: 40.22g
 Ingredients
 Calories
 Total Carbs (g)
 Fiber (g)
 Net Carbs (g)
 Protein (g)
 Fat (g)

Total per serving (/4)
569.56

10.41
4.28
6.14
38.39
40.23

Totals
2275.25
41.67
17.076
24.576
153.6
160.83

1 Roma Tomato
11
2.4
1.7
2.7
0.7
0.2

1/2 cup Sour Cream
223.5
3.6
0
3.6
2.5

22.6

1/4 cup sliced Pickled Jalapenos
6
2
0
2
0
0

1 cup shredded Mild Cheddar Cheese
443
4
0
4
29
37

1 Avocado
327
17
13
4
4
30

1 4 ounce can of Green Chiles
40
6

3
3
0
0

1/4 cup chopped Onion
28.75
1.75
0.38
1.38
0.2
2.25

1/4 cup Water
0
0
0
0
0
0

3/4 cup Red Enchilada Sauce
158
7
0
7
7
8

1 pound of Boneless Skinless Chicken Thigh
813
0
0
0
114.3
36.98

2 tablespoons Coconut Oil
235
0
0
0
0
29

Remember: everybody is different, and everyone's exact **macronutrient goals** are different.
Keto is a low carb, lean protein, high fat diet, and habitually followers of the keto diet will endeavor to hit their goals throughout a day's worth of eating, rather than trying to hit specific percentages for each meal.

Low carb meals can frequently be customized to meet your macro and flavor preferences. You could add more fat to this recipe by altering the amounts of ingredients such as cheese, avocado, or sour cream.

If you got a fatty coffee this morning and didn't want to surpass your fat for the day, you might try exchanging out the chicken thigh for a leaner chicken breast.
Change to what works for you, and be sure to share your best ideas with others.

58 Keto Chicken Enchilada Bowl

This Keto Chicken Enchilada Bowl is a low carb twist on a Mexican favored! It's SO stress-free to make, filling, and incredibly yummy!

- **Prep Time:** 22 minutes
- **Cook Time:** 32 minutes
- **Total Time:** 52 minutes
- **Yield:** 5 servings 1x

Ingredients
- 3tablespoons coconut oil (for searing chicken)
- 1 pound of boneless, skinless chicken thighs

- 3/4 cup red enchilada cheek (recipe from Low Carb Maven)
- 1/4 cup water
- 1/4 cup chopped onion
- 1– 4 oz can dice green chilies

Toppings (feel free to modify)
- 1 whole avocado, chopped
- 1 cup seared cheese (I used mild cheddar)
- 1/4 cup sliced pickled jalapenos
- 1/2 cup sour cream
- 1 Roma tomato, sautéed

Optional: serve over plain cauliflower rice (or Mexican cauliflower rice) for a complete meal!

Instructions

In a cooking pot or dutch oven over medium heat soften the coconut oil. Once hot, sear chicken thighs till lightly brown.

Decant in enchilada sauce, and water then put the extra onion and green chilies. Reduce heat to a simmer and cover. Cook chicken for 17-26 minutes or till chicken is tender and fully cooked through to at least 166 degrees internal temperature.

Carefully eliminate the chicken and put it onto a work surface.

Chop or shred chicken (your favorite), then add it back into the pot. Let the chicken simmer exposed for a further 11 minutes to absorb flavor and permit the sauce to lessen a little.

To serve, topped with avocado, cheese, jalapeno, sour cream, tomato, and any other chosen toppings. Feel free to make these to your taste.

Serve alone or over cauliflower rice; if needed, be sure to update your nutrition info as required.

Nutrition
- **Serving Size:** 1/4 recipe yield
- **Calories:** 568 Calories
- **Fat:** 40.22g
- **Carbohydrates:** 6.13g NET Carbs
- **Protein:** 38.39g

Hands-on 10 minutes Overall 20 minutes
Nutritional values (per serving)
Net carbs3.2 grams
Protein38.8 grams
Fat43.9 grams
Calories582 kcal
Calories from carbs **3%**, protein **29%**, fat **71%**

Total carbs**10.6**grams**Fiber7.5** grams

Total

carbs**10.6** gramsFiber**7.5** gramsSugars**1.3** grams   Saturated fat**10.2** gramsSodium**533** mg(23% RDA)Magnesium**80** mg(20% RDA)Potassium**1,032** mg(52% EMR)

Ingredients (make 2 servings)
· 2 boneless chicken breasts, skin on (286 g/ 11 oz)
· 6 thin-cut chopped bacon *or* 3 regular slices (91 g/ 3.3 oz)
· 1 large avocado, sliced (201 g/ 7.2 oz)
· 4 cups mixed leafy greens of choice (123 g/ 4.3 oz)
· 5tbsp. **Keto Ranch Dressing** (70 ml/ 3 fl oz) *or make* use dairy-free Ranch Dressing
· **<u>Ghee</u>** *or* duck fat for greasing
· salt and pepper, to taste

INSTRUCTIONS
1. Heat up the oven to 202 °C/ 400 °F. Begin by crisping up the chicken breasts. Spice the chicken body with salt and pepper from all sides. Grease a tiny skillet with ghee or duck fat. Place the chicken body, skin side down, on the hot pan.

2. Without moving it, roast the chicken on high until golden brown and crispy, for 5-7 minutes.

Then, change the chicken on the other side, cook for 32 seconds. Transfer the skillet into the oven.

3. Cook the chicken for 10-15 minutes. It's done when an instant-read thermometer inputted into the thickest part reads 74 °C/ 165 °F.

4. If you wish to bake the bacon in the oven, spread the slices over a baking sheet lined with parchment paper.

5. Bake for 11 minutes till crispy and golden brown. Alternatively, you can crisp up the bacon independently on a frying pan.

6. Once the chicken is boiled, convey to a cutting board and let it rest for 5 minutes.

7. Slice the avocado and the grilled chicken. Pull together the salad: start with the leafy greens and then add avocado, crispy bacon, and sliced chicken.

8. Topped the salad with 2 tablespoons of Ranch Dressing.

9. This salad is best served instantly. You could habitually keep some cooked chicken

and crisped up bacon in the fridge and reheat or use cold.

Ingredient nutritional breakdown (per serving)
Net carbs
Protein
Fat
Calories

Chicken, breast (with skin, raw)

0 g
29.7 g
13.2 g
245 kcal

Bacon, streaky (high-fat content), organic

0 g
6.2 g
11.3 g
126 kcal

Avocado, fresh

1.9 g
2 g
14.7 g

160 kcal

Lettuce, mixed leaf salad

0.8 g
0.8 g
0.1 g
8 kcal

Ranch Dressing built with Avocado Oil (Primal Kitchen)

0.7 g
0 g
4.5 g
42 kcal

Total per serving

3.1 g
38.7 g
43.8 g
581 kcal
Ingredient nutritional breakdown (per serving)
Net carbs
Protein
Fat
Calories

Chicken, breast (with skin, raw)

0 g
29.7 g
13.2 g
245 kcal

Bacon, streaky (high-fat content), organic

0 g
6.2 g
11.3 g
126 kcal

Avocado, fresh

1.9 g
2 g
14.7 g
160 kcal

Lettuce, mixed leaf salad

0.8 g
0.8 g
0.1 g
8 kcal

Ranch Dressing made with Avocado Oil (Primal Kitchen)

0.7 g
0 g
4.5 g
42 kcal

Total per serving

3.1 g
38.7 g
43.8 g
581 kcal

59   5-INGREDIENT   LOW   CARB CHEESECAKE RECIPE

This 5-Ingredient Low Carb Cheesecake Recipe is an excellent choice when everyone else is eating regular cheesecake, though you're trying to stay low carb or keto! These mini cheesecakes are creamy and spicy with merely 3g carbs per serving.

Individuals regularly think cheesecake is a no-no when sticking to a healthy eating plan. Rich and indulgent, normal cheesecake is one of the most decadent tasting desserts.

Well, so is this cheesecake. The only thing it's missing is carbs, and I have said it you won't even miss them! (Who requires crust on cheesecake, anyway?)

I've experimented a lot with diverse ratios of cream cheese to eggs, and I've also tried this recipe adding in other ingredients, similar to sour cream and heavy cream.

In the final analysis, I think this kind comes closest to typical cheesecake in its creamy texture. I like keeping a batch of these stored in the fridge to enjoy as a quick snack or dessert throughout the week.

WHAT IS THE BEST LOW CARB DESSERT?

The finest low carb dessert is, of course, a matter of individual disposition. To me, it is, without a bit of doubt, cheesecake! This is because I feel low carb keto cheesecake tastes more like the regular version than most other desserts do.

Another pint why cheesecake is the best low carb dessert is that it's stress-free to change a common recipe for cheesecake into a low carb recipe.

The two leading sources of carbs in cheesecake come from the crust and the sweetener, so if you could swap out low carb alternatives for both, you'll quickly have a treat that's much lower in carbs.

BEST LOW CARB CHEESECAKE
The finest low carb cheesecake is one that has a rich, creamy texture with an impeccable sweetness level. As an additional benefit, it should be easy to make!

My 5-constituents: Low Carb Cheesecake Recipe is as captivating as it is stress-free to whip up, and is very close to normal cheesecake in both flavor and texture.

LOW CARB CHEESECAKE INGREDIENTS

This recipe has merely five ingredients, and you normally have all or most of them on hand already:
· Cream cheese
· Eggs
· Stevia/erythritol blend
· Vanilla extract
· Almond extract

LOW CARB CHEESECAKE CRUST:
I very much love cheesecake without crust; I think the cheesecake itself is the best part! However, if you wish to make a crust for your cheesecake, an excellent ingredient to use as the fundamental is nut meal or flour, similar to almond, pecan, hazelnut, etc.

I have an excellent recipe for Low Carb Pumpkin Spice Cheesecake for you, An Edible Mosaic, which you can modify to use in these mini cheesecakes if you want.

HOW TO CREATE THE BEST LOW CARB CHEESECAKE:
For this recipe, I begin with softened cream cheese, but note that this doesn't mean hot cream cheese. I let the cream cheese get to room temperature, and then I soften it for just some seconds in the microwave, since it's

very calm to beat until smooth. After that, I blend in the remaining ingredients (eggs, stevia, and vanilla and almond extracts), pour the pound into a lined muffin tray, and cook for about 15 to 22 minutes. It's so easy; there's no need even to use a water bath with this recipe!

LOW CARB CHEESECAKE NUTRITION
What ARE THE NUMBERS OF CARBS IN LOW CARB CHEESECAKE?

Per serving, this low carb cheesecake recipe contains 3g carbs.

HOW MANY ARE CALORIES IN SUGAR-FREE CHEESECAKE?
Each serving of this sugar-free cheesecake has 181kcals.
CAN YOU CONSUME CHEESECAKE ON A KETO DIET?

Yes! Cheesecake is a splendid choice when you're on a keto diet, and you want something to satisfy your sweet tooth. Because it's not very low in fat, this cheesecake is very satiating.
KETO CHEESECAKE:

Keto cheesecake is lean in carbs and high in fat to make you maintain a state of nutritional ketosis.

It usually uses sweeteners such as stevia and erythritol, and it typically has a nut-based crust or no crust at all, such as my 5-Ingredient Low Carb **Cheesecake Recipe**.

You could serve it as-is, or with a drizzle of sugar-free caramel, a sprinkle of stevia-sweetened chocolate chips, or with some raspberries or blackberries on top.

5-Ingredient Low Carb Cheesecake Recipe:
This 5-Ingredient Lean Carb Cheesecake Recipe is a fantastic choice when everyone else is eating regular cheesecake; moreover, you're trying to stay low carb or keto!
These mini cheesecakes are tasty and very rich, with just 3g carbs per serving.

Ingredients
· 8 oz full-fat cream cheese softened
· 2 large eggs
· 1 1/2 teaspoons granulated stevia/erythritol mix
· 1/4 teaspoon pure vanilla extract
· 1/4 teaspoon pure almond extract

Instructions

1. Preheat oven to 326F; line 5 muffin wells with liners.
2. Beat the cream cheese until smooth; however, beat in the eggs and all remaining components.
3. Pour the pound into the prepared muffin tray and bake till the cheesecakes start to puff, though are still wobbly in the crux, about 15 to 22 minutes (be careful not to over-bake!).
4. Cool to the room temperature and later chill for 2 hours before serving.
5. Store leftovers enclosed in the fridge for up to 1 week.

Helpful Tips
Net Carbs: 2g per serving
Nutrition
Calories: 185kcal | Carbohydrates: 2g | Protein: 4g | Fat: 18g | Saturated Fat: 10g | Cholesterol: 116mg | Sodium: 172mg | Potassium: 87mg | Sugar: 1g | Vitamin A: 706IU | Calcium: 55mg | Iron: 0.6mg

57 Breakfast: Green Shakshuka

Traditional shakshuka, an Arabic version of poached eggs in tomatoes, peppers, and onions, is somewhat low in carbs, though, it's not appropriate if you're following a strict keto diet. Fortuitously, it's easy to make this delicious one-skillet dish keto-friendly: use low-carb veggies, like zucchini and spinach.

Yields: 5 servings
 Preparation time: 12 minutes
 Cooking time: 16 minutes
Ingredients
 3 tablespoons (32g) ghee or other healthy cooking fat
 1 clove garlic, minced
 1 medium (120g) green bell pepper, sautéed
 ½ small (35g) yellow onion, sliced
 1 minute (150g) zucchini, cut into ½-inch (1-cm) cubes
 ½ cup (120g) canned diced tomatoes
 ¼ teaspoon ground coriander
 ½ teaspoon paprika
 1/8 teaspoon cayenne pepper
 Salt and ground black pepper
 3 cups (90g) fresh spinach
 5 large eggs
 1 tablespoon (4g) fresh cilantro or parsley, cut
 ½ teaspoon ground cumin.
Directions
- In a wide skillet oiled with ghee, cook the onion over medium-high heat for 5 to 8 minutes, until lightly browned.

- Add garlic, green pepper, and zucchini. Cook for about 3 minutes, stirring occasionally.
- Add tomatoes, cumin, paprika, coriander, cayenne pepper, sea salt, and black pepper — Cook for about 6 minutes, or until the vegetables are tender.
- Put the spinach and cook for 2 minutes, until wilted.
- Use a spatula to make 5 wells in the mixture. Break 1 egg into every well, and cook up until the whites are opaque and the yolks are still runny. Take away from the heat.
- Garnish with the cilantro. Serve instantly, or store it for up to 2 days (without the fried eggs).

Per Serving
Fat: 25.4g
Protein: 16.3g
Carbohydrate: 12.6g
Calories: 338
Macronutrient ratio: Calories from carbs vary (10 percent), protein (20 percent), fat (70 percent)

60 Lunch: Ratatouille Soup

: Some soups, similar to this delicate version of ratatouille, are best prepared on the stovetop, with ingredients added gradually. It features pesto and fresh herbs, which have volatile oils—to preserve their flavors, they should be added at the tail end of the cooking process.

Yields: 5 servings
Preparation time: 10 minutes
Cooking time: 25 minute
Ingredients
Soup:
2 tablespoons (32g) ghee or other healthy cooking fat
1 small (110g) yellow onion, sliced
2 cloves garlic, minced
1 medium (120g) green bell pepper, diced
1 medium (121g) yellow or orange bell pepper, diced
2 cups (480ml) vegetable or chicken stock
1 medium (200g) zucchini, chopped
1 medium (250g) eggplant, chopped
2 cups (480ml) water
1 teaspoon dried oregano
14.1 ounces (400g) canned diced tomatoes
2 tablespoons (30g) Red Pesto
Salt and ground black pepper
Topping:

6 oz (170g) fresh mozzarella di bufala
6 tablespoons (90ml) extra-virgin olive oil
Fresh basil

Directions

- Heat a skillet oiled with ghee over medium heat. Add the onion and cook it over medium-high heat for 5 to 8 minutes, until lightly browned.
- Add the garlic, peppers, zucchini, and eggplant. Cook for 1 to 3 minutes, stirring constantly.
- Add the oregano, tomatoes, stock, and water. Bring to heat, and cook over medium heat for about 16 minutes, or until the vegetables remain tender.
- Take off the heat. Use a spoon to move half of the vegetables to a bowl and set aside.
- Make use of dipping blender to purée the leftover vegetables. Place the remaining vegetables back into the pot and put the pesto. Stir and season with salt and pepper.
- To serve, put the soup into bowls and top with a piece of fresh mozzarella cheese.

Drizzle each bowl with a tablespoon (16 ml) of olive oil and garnish with basil leaves. To store, let it cool and chill it in an airtight container for up to 5 days or cool for up to 3 months (minus the toppings).

Per Serving (About 1½ Cups/360ml)

Fat: 29.1g

Protein: 7g

Carbohydrate: 11.9g

Calories: 338

Macronutrient ratio: Calories coming from carbs (10 percent), protein (11 percent), fat (79 percent)